Sondes Laajimi
Haifa Bradai
Nabil Chebbi

Simulation-based learning at the Faculty of Medicine in Sousse

Sondes Laajimi
Haifa Bradai
Nabil Chebbi

Simulation-based learning at the Faculty of Medicine in Sousse

ScienciaScripts

Imprint

Any brand names and product names mentioned in this book are subject to trademark, brand or patent protection and are trademarks or registered trademarks of their respective holders. The use of brand names, product names, common names, trade names, product descriptions etc. even without a particular marking in this work is in no way to be construed to mean that such names may be regarded as unrestricted in respect of trademark and brand protection legislation and could thus be used by anyone.

Cover image: www.ingimage.com

This book is a translation from the original published under ISBN 978-620-6-71834-5.

Publisher:
Sciencia Scripts
is a trademark of
Dodo Books Indian Ocean Ltd. and OmniScriptum S.R.L publishing group

120 High Road, East Finchley, London, N2 9ED, United Kingdom
Str. Armeneasca 28/1, office 1, Chisinau MD-2012, Republic of Moldova, Europe
Printed at: see last page
ISBN: 978-620-8-12989-7

Background: Healthcare simulation has become a crucial teaching technique in various medical disciplines. This approach, using virtual reality or standardised patients to reproduce clinical scenarios, has proved essential in preparing medical students for high-risk situations, ensuring the safe and effective management of critical patients through the acquisition of technical skills, teamwork and the ability to manage exceptional scenarios. The aims of this study were to assess students' theoretical knowledge before and after the simulation-based training (SBT) of the "Advanced Cardiopulmonary Resuscitation (CPR)" module, to evaluate their technical and non-technical skills, and to describe their satisfaction. **Methods**: A pre-experimental study conducted at the Faculty of Medicine aimed to objectively assess the impact of FBS on the theoretical knowledge, technical skills and non-technical skills of graduating medical students during their advanced CPR training **Results**: We demonstrated that FBS was highly valued by the learners and led to significant improvements in their theoretical knowledge. There was a positive correlation between the pre-test and post-test scores, with a correlation coefficient of r = 0.474, p < 0.0001, r^2 = 0,245. For technical skills, 69.8% improved their external cardiac massage (ECM) technique by the day of the test, while 14 (16.3%) showed a decline (p < 0.001). In addition, "non-technical skills" (NTS) were assessed using the Non-Technical Skills in Anaesthesia (NTSA) score among these students, 85 (89.5%) improved their scores, while 10 (10.5%) maintained their initial scores (p < 0.001). At the end of the training sessions, a strong statistically significant correlation was found between the sum of the post-test scores, the ANTS score, the cardiac massage score and the final score of the "ECOS" simulated practical examination (r = 0.762, p < 0.001, r^2 = 0,581). Student satisfaction was assessed; overall, student impressions were mainly excellent in more than 50% of responses.
Conclusion: The study's contribution to the growing body of evidence supporting the integration of simulation-based learning into early medical education is particularly noteworthy. Simulation can accelerate skill acquisition and improve the transition of knowledge and confidence in the face of critical real-life scenarios.
Key words: Simulation, Medical students, Education, Undergraduate, cardiopulmonary resuscitation

Simulation is considered to be one of the key teaching techniques in the health sciences in several fields. The French Haute Autorité de Santé (HAS) defined healthcare simulation in 2012 as "the use of equipment, virtual reality or a standardised patient to reproduce healthcare situations or environments, with the aim of teaching diagnostic and therapeutic procedures, rehearsing medical processes and concepts, or decision-making by a healthcare professional or team of professionals"(1).

Simulation in healthcare has become necessary in the teaching of so-called "high-risk" medical disciplines. The safety and innocuousness of managing a patient's critical condition depends on learning technical and therapeutic gestures according to a management algorithm and on good interaction between the different team members involved(2).

Simulation can reproduce an exceptional situation ad infinitum, offers risk-free learning for both patient and learner, and enables cognitive, technical and human aspects to be worked on. It is associated with an increase in knowledge and skills among learners and helps to improve patient prognosis (3).

To assess the impact of simulation-based training, the HAS recommends using the Kirkpatrick model. This model divides the effectiveness of the teaching intervention into 4 levels, depending on the behavioural changes made by the learners. Each level is constructed from the information provided at the preceding levels (4).

In continuing education, simulation in healthcare is beginning to gain ground in France; currently, in initial medical training, the development of simulation has led to the creation of objective and structured clinical examinations (OSCEs) for medical students, which are a form of simulation by putting students in situations that enable them not only to learn, but also to be assessed summatively(5).

The new reform of medical studies, introduced at the Faculty of Medicine in Sousse in 2016, has adopted a competency-based, learner-centred study programme using new active learning methods and resources such as simulation, case-based learning (CBL) and team-based learning (TBL). These new learning methods need to be evaluated.

CPR "advanced cardiopulmonary resuscitation" is a block designed for DCEM3 students. It was recently introduced during the 2020-2021 academic year as a module to be taught by simulation (Appendix 1). Through this study, we carried out an evaluative approach structured according to the Kirkpatrick model (levels 1 and 2) of the pedagogical contribution of this learning method, taught at the Faculty of Medicine in Sousse and dedicated to DCEM 3 students in the 2022-2023 academic year.

The objectives of our study :

To assess the level of theoretical knowledge and technical and non-technical skills of DCEM3 students before and after simulation-based learning of the "Advanced CPR" module.

-describe the levels of student satisfaction with simulation training in the "Advanced CPR" module

I. *Type of study:*

This is a pre-experimental study that took place at the Faculty of Medicine in Sousse, involving the DCEM3 level in terms of CPR during the 2022-2023 academic year.

II. *Study population :*

We included in our study all DCEM 3 students who were present during their Bloc CPR in the academic year 2022-2023.

The students were divided by the faculty administration into 5 groups, each group consisting of around 40 students divided into two training centres

For each group, we carried out hybrid simulation training using low-fidelity mannequins.

1. **Inclusion criteria :**

-All medical students enrolled in DCEM 3 at the Sousse Faculty of Medicine

-students who applied for CPR training

2. **Exclusion criteria :**

Students who are absent for the post-test, pre-test or exam

3. **Non-inclusion criteria :**

- students not authorised to sit the CPR exam

III. *The course :*

The training took place according to a predefined programme, essentially in the form of practical simulation workshops spread over two days.

All students took a pre- and post-test to assess their level of knowledge.

A draw was made beforehand to identify two groups for which non-technical procedures were assessed using the ANTS score and a technical procedure, external cardiac massage (ECM), was assessed. The topics taught were Workshop 1: Basic Life Support (BLS) and defibrillation.

Workshop 2: Management of a critically ill patient using the ABCDE approach.

Workshop 3: Airway management.

Workshop 4: ECG monitoring and rhythm recognition/algorithm for tachycardia and bradycardia Workshop 5: Shockable rhythms and resuscitation after cardiopulmonary arrest.

Workshop 6: Non-shockable rhythms and the decision to stop resuscitation.

Workshop 7: special circumstances in the event of an RTA

For each group

<u>STEP 1:</u>

<u>The day of the training</u> Welcome, reminder of the objectives of the CPR module, the objectives of the various practical workshops; how the day will be run.

The training began with a pre-test in the form of multiple-choice questions (MCQs) (see appendix 2). It consisted of 15 questions relating to the main objectives of the training.

This stage is used to assess the theoretical pre-requisites of students whose theoretical support was previously sent to the UVT platform.

<u>STAGE 2: This</u> corresponds to the actual training in the form of various practical workshops (see appendix 3).

An assessment at the beginning of the training (Workshop 1) of a selected technical skill, which was External Cardiac Massage (ECM), only for the groups selected at random (see appendix 4). The non-technical skills were assessed according to the "ANTS" score during the training course during the "Case-Teach" simulation scenarios (n°1, 2, 3, 4) in which the learner plays the role of a "Team Leader" in a team effort to manage a patient in critical condition (see appendix 5).

STEP 3: At the end of the day's training, we assessed the student's learning by means of a theory test (Post-Test).

A practical examination (Clinical Scenario) in the form of an OSCE station for all students present at the examination We assessed the non-technical procedures in the randomly selected groups according to the ANTS score, as well as the technical procedure, which was MCE.

Finally, we ended with an evaluation of learner satisfaction with this simulation-based learning method, using a satisfaction grid.

IV. *Course duration and locations :*

The average duration of the training was eight (08) hours and took place in parallel in two simulation training centres:

*CESIM of the Sousse Faculty of Medicine

 *SAMU 03 training centre

V. *The measuring instrument :*

3 measuring instruments were chosen and validated according to Kirkpatrick's level of assessment:

The Kirkpatrick model has defined a training evaluation model based on 4 levels of evaluation (see Appendix 6)

1. The first level, called "reaction", is used to assess learner satisfaction. A learner satisfaction evaluation grid provided to students at the end of the session; grid validated at institutional level (CESIM). (See Annex 7).

2. The second level measures 'learning' in terms of the knowledge, skills and attitudes acquired during their learning experiences.

A self-completed medical questionnaire (inspired by the ESL

questionnaire on the ERC platform) to assess learners' pre-requisite knowledge (Pre-test).

This questionnaire contains 14 questions, of which approximately 30% represent taxonomic level 3.

An assessment grid for technical and non-technical skills:

A massage technique assessment grid

RESCAPE-CM in terms of MCE in older children and adapted it to adults. The cardiac massage technique was evaluated in two randomly selected groups (D and E), based on 13 criteria, with each criterion scored on one point.

**These criteria were : massage method suitable for an adult, positioning the victim on a hard surface, correct frequency, compression ration; compression/ventilation ratio 30/2, correct depression of the thorax, minimising the interruption time of cardiac massage, the hand is correctly placed on the thorax, the fingers do not rest on the thorax, lateral positioning in relation to the victim, arms outstretched with elbows locked, depression of the thorax perpendicular to the axis of the body, and the heel of the hand does not come off the thorax during the relaxation phase.

S An assessment grid for non-technical skills: the "ANTS" score: Anesthesia Non Technical Skills.

3. the third level, called "transfer", to evaluate changes and modifications in the behaviour of learners in their working environment

4. the fourth level, called "result", identifies the impact of simulation training on patient care.

It was not possible to assess levels 3 and 4 during our study, as the CPR block was not associated with a practical placement allowing us to observe our learners in their work environment.

VI. *Data analysis :*

The data was analysed using SPSS For the descriptive study: the normality of the distribution of the variables was verified using the Kolmogorov-Smirnov test. Continuous variables were expressed according to a normal distribution by their means and standard deviation and discontinuous variables by their proportions.

For the univariate analysis, means were compared using the Student's t-test and the test for independent samples, and percentages were compared using the Chi-square test. Pearson correlation was used to look for correlations between the continuous variables of interest.

The ANOVA test was used to compare the average marks between the different groups of students.

A $p < 0.05$ was considered significant.

VII. *Ethical considerations :*

Completion of the questionnaire was subject to the written and informed consent of the candidates and to individual and institutional authorisation.

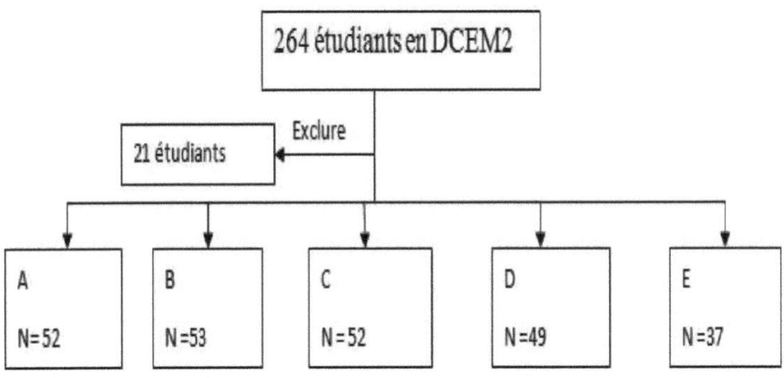

Figure 1: Study flow chart

A. <u>Descriptive study</u>

I. <u>*Characteristics of the general population*</u>

This cohort of 5th year medical students comprises 264 students divided into 5 groups

21 were excluded from this analysis, we included 243 students

1. <u>Breakdown of students by gender :</u>

There were 192 women (73%) and 71 men (27%).

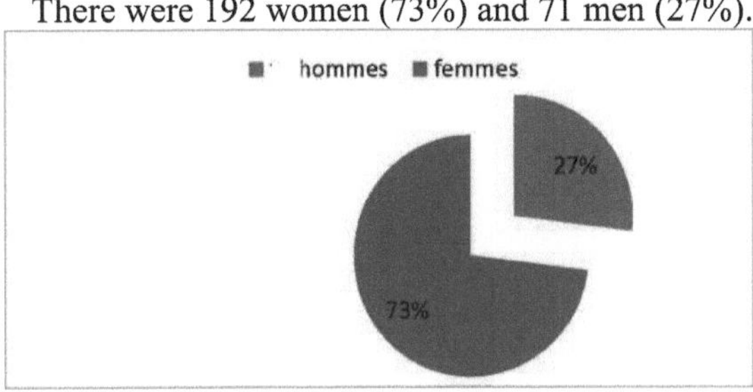

Figure 2: Breakdown of students by gender

2. <u>Breakdown of students by age :</u>

The average age of our population was 23.6 (±0.7) with extremes ranging from 22-28.

3. **Breakdown of students by group :**

Groups A, B and C have between 52 and 53 students except group D which has 49 students and group E which has 37 students.

Table I: Breakdown by group

Group name	Number (N)
A	52
B	53
C	52
D	49
E	37

II. *Assessment of learning (Kirkpatrick level 2)*

1. **Evaluation of theoretical training ("knowledge" assessment) before and after the course**

a. Pre- and post-test notes

We gave each group a self-completed questionnaire before and after the training day. This questionnaire comprises 14 questions with taxonomic levels ranging from 1 to 3 according to the specification table. We gave each student a score out of 20.

The median pre-test score was 9.5 [7.75 - 12],

the median post-test score was 13 [14.75 - 11.5].

This difference was statistically significant ($p < 0.0001$).

At the end of the CPR training day, 205 (84.4%) of the students had improved their grade, 26 (10.7%) had regressed and 12 (4.5%) had the same initial grade.

The scores for the different groups are summarised in the table below.

Group	Median [IIQ]		
	Pre-test	Post test	p
A	14 [12,31 -15,37]	14,25 [12,62 -15,5]	0.07
B	9,6 [8,3 - 11,18]	12,75 [11,68 -15]	0.005
C	9 [11,5 - 8]	13,75[11,68 - 15,56]	0.001
D	9 [6,9 - 10]	13 [11,5 - 14,56]	0.001
E	7,75 [6,12 - 9]	11[10 - 12,75]	0.012
All groups	9,5 [7,75 - 12]	13 [14,75 - 11,5]	**<0.0001**

b. Scores questions at taxonomy level 3

Four questions presented a level 3 taxonomy in the form of a multiple-choice MCQ or a QROC. These were questions 2, 8, 11 and 14.

For question 2: **in the pre-test, 190 (72%) of the students got a full mark.**

In the post-test, we noted an improvement, with **235 (96.7%) receiving a full mark,** although 9 (3.3%) received a zero.

We noted that 49 (20.2%) improved their score, and **82% of those who had scored zero in the pre-test improved their score,** although 4 (1.6%) regressed.

The improvement in the mark for question 2 led to an improvement in the mark for the post-test, with a statistically significant difference (p=0.003).

For question 8: **in the pre-test, 126 (51.8%)** students scored > average, including 42 (17.3%) who scored full marks, compared with 117 (48.14%) who scored below average, including 109 (44.9%) who scored zero.

In the post-test, 77 (31.7%) obtained a full mark, of which 168 (69.2%) had a mark > the average. 72 (29.6%), however, obtained a zero. An improvement was noted in 91 (37.4%) of cases. Knowing that the improvement in the score on question 8 significantly influenced the improvement in the score on the post-test (p=0.003), and that approximately 25% of the participants had a zero on the pre- and post-tests.

For question 11: **in the pre-test**, only 39 (16%) students scored full marks, with **54 (22.2%)** scoring >average; 189 (77.8%) students scored zero.

In the post-test, 71 (26.9%) received a full mark compared with 163 (67.1%) who received a zero.

75 (30.8%) scored above average. Knowing that 54% kept the zero mark in the pre- and post-test. We noted an improvement in only 62 students (25.5%).

The non-improvement of the score for question 11, which deals with the "treatment of poorly tolerated tachycardia", is significantly correlated with the non-improvement of the score for the "treatment of poorly tolerated tachycardia".

post test (p=0.007).

For question 14: **in the pre-test, only 2 students (0.8%) received a full mark,** while 82 (33.9%) received a zero and 166 (68.3%) received a mark below average.

In the post-test we noted an improvement in 126 (52.1%) of the students; **34 (14%) had a full mark** with 132 (54.3%) who had a mark > average.

Table III: Level III question scores

Question	Full note N (%)	Zero N (%)	Below average N (%)	Above average N (%)
Q2 pre	190 (72)	53 (21,8)	-	
Q2 post	235 (96,7)	9 (3,3)		
8 meadow	42 (17,3)	109 (44,9)	117 (41	126 (51,8)
Q8 post	77 (31,7)	72 (29,6)	75 (30,8)	168 (69,2)
Q11 pre	39 (16)	189 (77,8)	189 (77	54 (22,2)
Q11 post	71 (26 ,9)	163 (67,1)	168 (69,2)	75 (30,8)
Q14 pre	2 (0,8)	82 (33,9)	166 (68	77 (31,6)
Q14 post	34 (14)	52 (21,4)	111 (45,6)	132 (54,3)

2. Assessment of technical and non-technical learning (assessment of "knowing how to do/savoir être") before and after the training course

We drew two groups at random D (N=49) and group
E (N= 37) to assess technical and non-technical skills

a. <u>Assessment of cardiac massage technique</u>

A first mark was awarded for a first pass during the learning session of the group concerned and the second during the final exam.

Cardiac massage is graded according to a grid with a full score of 13

The median initial score was 11 [9 - 12], the median final score was 12 [10.75 - 13].

We noted that 12 (14%) of the two groups had an excellent technique from the outset (from the start of their training day); and that 60 (69.8%) improved their cardiac massage technique on the day of the examination, while 14 (16.3%) regressed in this skill.

Figure 3: Evolution of the cardiac massage technique score during the

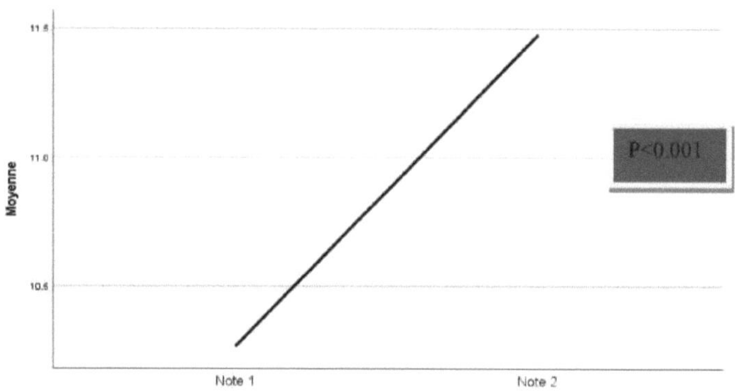

b. <u>Assessment of learning of non-technical skills</u>

Among the two groups drawn at random we have the "non-technical skills" by the ANTS score, the first average at the beginning of the training was 6.4 (±1.7), the average retained on the day of the exam (simulation scenario) was 10.2 (±2.5). 85 (89.5%) of these students improved their marks and 10 (10.5%) had the same mark as at the beginning of the training.

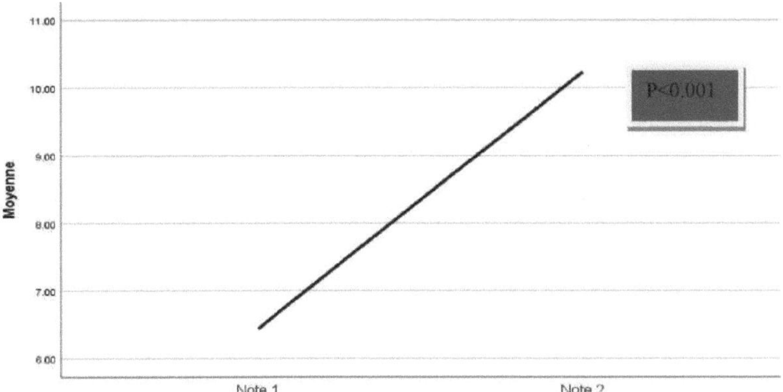

Figure 4: Changes in ANTS score during simulation training

3. <u>Assessment of simulated practice (simulation scenario)</u>

At the end of the training sessions, the 5 groups of students take a practical exam in the form of "ECOS" stations, where each student takes the exam as a "first responder" or as a "team member".

At each visit, the students belonging to the two groups drawn at random were assessed on their technical and non-technical skills using the same grids used during the first days of training.

However, all the groups of students took the final exam in the form of simulated practice, a simulation scenario during which the students were assessed on their knowledge, skills and attitudes according to a well-coded grid (see appendix).

The median score was 16 [15 - 18], and the scores for the

different groups are summarised in the table below.

Table IV: Simulation score as a function of group

Group	Median [IIQ]
A	16 [15 - 18]
B	15,75 [14,75 - 17]
C	17 [16 - 18]
D	17 [15 - 18,5]
E	15 [14 - 18]

III. *Assessment of student satisfaction (Kirkpatrick level 1)*

At the end of the CPR module, we assessed student satisfaction using an evaluation grid validated by the institution, which includes 44 items relating to the introduction to the module and the documents provided, the equipment, the quality of the scenarios, the debriefing and the instructors.

We have eliminated all incorrectly completed or incomplete forms,

211 forms were collected.

The general impression of the students was quite excellent, in more than 50% of the responses.

Around 77% found the documents provided before the training session good or even excellent. As for the general assessment of the simulation room, around 88% found it good to excellent.

87% of students rated the script's ability to convey attitudes and behaviours as good to excellent.

86% of the students considered the debriefing at the end of the scenario to be constructive and over 90% appreciated the overall quality of the debriefing.

The general quality of the instructors' work was considered good to excellent by more than 91% of the students.

The responses to this questionnaire are summarised in the table below.

Table V: Assessment of student satisfaction with the CPR module

Element	Score given by student (N = 211(P))				
	Inadequate	Insufficient	Suitable	Good	Excellent
The introduction					
Document to read	1 (0,5)	13 (6,2)	35 (16,6)	91 (43,1	71 (33,6)
Introduction	3 (1,4)	5 (2,4)	29 (13,7)	92 (43,6)	82 (38,9)
Revision of the video trigger	16 (7,6)	13 (6,2)	33 (15,6)	76 (36)	73 (34,6)
Simulator orientation	1 (0,5)	9 (4,3)	20 (9,5)	86 (40,8)	95 (45)
Equipment and environment					
General organisation of the simulation room	2 (0,9)	2 (0,9)	16 (7,6)	77 (36,5)	114 (54)
Mannequins	4 (1,9)	0	16 (7,6)	88 (41,7)	103 (48,8)
Patient monitor	3 (1,4)	0	14 (6,6)	76 (36)	118 (55,9)
Checklist	1 (0,5)	3 (1,4)	28 (13,3)	74 (35,1)	105 (49,8)
Medication provided	3 (1,4)	9 (4,3)	24 (11,4)	74 (35,1)	101 (47,9)
Audiovisual equipment	9 (4,3)	10 (4,7)	23 (10,9)	63 (29,9)	106 (50,2)
General realism of the simulation environment	3 (1,4)	3 (1,4)	18 (8,5)	78 (37)	109 (51,7)
Scenarios					
Realistic scenarios	1 (0,5)	6 (2,8)	14 (6,6)	79 (37,4)	111 (52,6)
Realistic visual cues	4 (1,9)	6 (2,8)	25 (11,8)	84 (39,8)	92 (43,6)
Realistic sound cues	3 (1,4)	5 (2,4)	28 (13,3)	81 (38,4)	94 (44,5)
Realistic tactile cues	1 (0,5)	9 (4,3)	29 (13,7)	73 (34,6)	99 (46,9)
Realism of the actors or patient partners in the scenarios	0	3 (1,4)	27 (12,8)	74 (35,1)	107 (50,7)
Ability of the scenario to demonstrate technical skills	0	5 (2,4)	21 (10)	76 (36)	109 (51,7)
Ability of the scenario to highlight attitudes and behaviours	0	5 (2,4)	18 (8,5)	82 (38,9)	106 (50,2)

Overall quality of scripts	0	3 (1,4)	16 (7,6)	83 (39,3)	109 (51,7)
Debriefing					
Clarified a number of specific points	3 (1,4)	3 (1,4)	21 (10)	84 (39,8)	100 (47,4)
Provided constructive feedback	2 (0,9)	4 (1,9)	23 (10,9)	84 (39,8)	98 (46,4)
Reviewed the technical skills demonstrated	2 (0,9)	1 (0,5)	21 (10)	82 (38,9)	105 (49,8)
Reviewed the attitudes and behaviours demonstrated	2 (0,9)	3 (1,4)	18 (8,5)	79 (37,4)	109 (51,7)
Overall quality of the debriefing	2 (0,9)	4 (1,9)	12 (5,7)	84 (39,8)	109 (51,7)
Instructors					
Instructors have created a welcoming learning environment	3 (1,4)	3 (1,4)	13 (6,2)	71 (33,6)	121 (57,3)
The instructors facilitated the debriefing	1 (0,5)	3 (1,4)	19 (9)	60 (28,4)	128 (60,7)
The instructors were able to create links between the scenarios	1 (0,5	1 (0,5)	18 (8,5	64 (30,3	127 (30,3)
Enthusiastic instructors	1 (0,5)	1 (0,5)	22 (10,4)	56 (26,5)	131 (62,1)
Overall quality of the instructors' work	3 (1,4	0	17 (8,1	62 (29,4	129 (61,1)
Overall impression of the CPR module	1 (0,5)	4 (1,9)	11 (5,2)	79 (37,4)	116 (55)

Among the written comments; two students cited that the document provided was too long, with one citing that the document did not cover all the objectives. Other students, 7, considered the training programme to be too fast-paced.

To improve the way CPR sessions are run, our students suggest :

+ Improved mannequins for VA management and cardiac massage, with the addition of visual and sound effects.

+ More scenarios, more rehearsals, more practice which was limited by the time constraint

+ Taking the ECG/rhythm disorder workshop further

+ Spread the CPR learning module over 3 days

+ Have printed protocols and PowerPoint presentations available,

+ Record videos of sessions and post them on YouTube

B. <u>Analytical study</u>

I. <u>*Univariate study*</u>

1. <u>Correlation between post-test score and simulated practice score</u>

There was a positive correlation between the post-test score and the simulation score, with a correlation coefficient r =0.237, p<0.0001, r^2 =0.056.

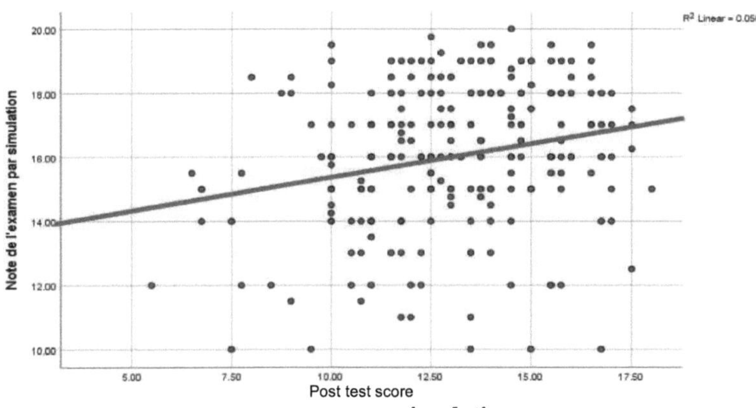

Figure 5: Scatter plot of post-test scores versus simulation scores.

2. <u>Correlation between pre-test score and post-test score</u>

There was a positive correlation between the pre-test score and the post-test score, with a correlation coefficient r =0.474, p<0.0001, r2 =0.245.

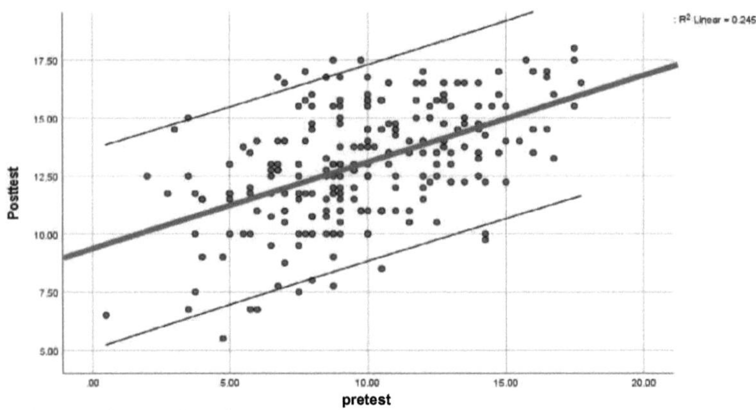

Figure 6: Scatter plot of post-test scores versus pre-test scores

3. <u>Comparison of groups</u>

a. <u>Sex</u>

There was no statistically significant difference between men and women in terms of improvement in the level of learning of the various skills (this is summarised in the table below).

Table VI: Comparison by gender

Type	Pre-test	Post-test	Simulation
Men	9,25	12,62	16
Woman	9,5	13	16
P	0,582	0,402	0,247

b. <u>Group running order</u>

We found a statistically significant difference ($p < 0.05$) when comparing the scores on the different assessments in relation to the order in which the groups were placed.

groups. Group A seemed to have the highest scores, compared with the
rest of the groups.

Table VII: Comparison by group

Group	Pre-test	Post-test	Simulation
A	14	14,25	16
B	9,62	12,75	15,75
C	9	13,75	17
D	9	13	17
E	7,75	11	15
p	<0,0001	<0,0001	0,012

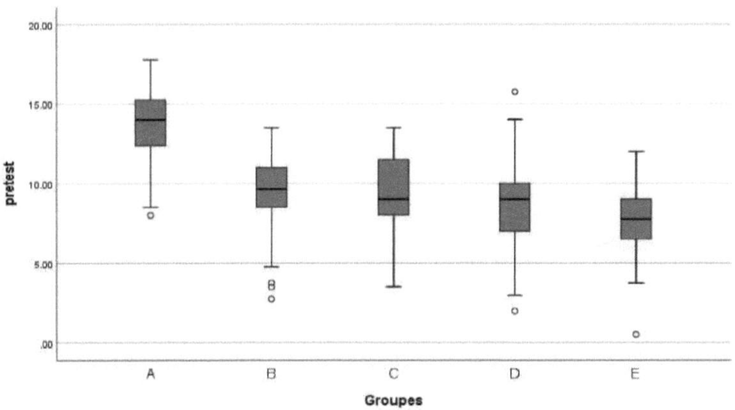

Figure 7: Mouse box plot of pre-test scores by group

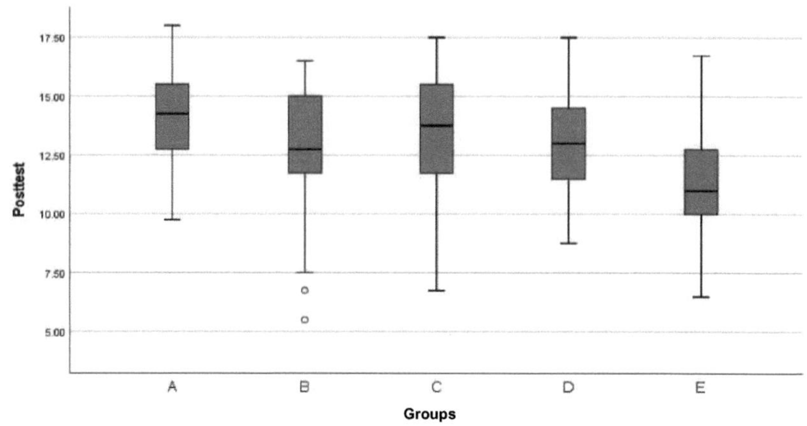

Figure 8: Box plot of post-test scores by group

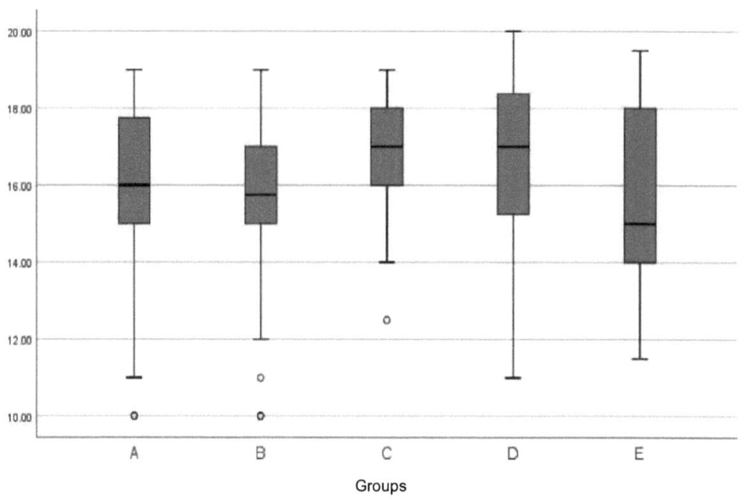

Figure 9: Moustache box of Simulation scores by group

Of the students who did not improve their marks in the post-test, 157 (97.4%) did not improve their marks in question 2, 120 (84.2%) did not improve their marks in question 8, 146 (92.1%) did not improve their marks in question 11, and 115 (7/1%) improved their marks in question 14.

Non-improvement in the learning curve for questions at taxonomic level 3 had a negative impact on improvement in the level of theoretical knowledge, with a statistically significant difference (p=0.000).

Table VIII: Influence of questions with taxonomy level 3 on the development of theoretical knowledge

Variable		Post-test score		P
		Improvement	No improvement	
Q2	Improvement	48 (23,4)	1 (2,6)	0,003
	No improvement	157 (76,6)	37 (97,4)	
Q8	Improvement	85 (41,5)	6 (15,8)	0,003
	No improvement	120 (58,5)	32 (84,2)	
Q11	Improvement	59 (28,8)	3 (7,9)	0,007
	No improvement	146 (71,2)	35 (92,1)	
Q14	Improvement	115 (56,4)	11 (28,9)	0,002
	No improvement	89 (43,6)	27 (71,1)	
Sum	Improvement	150 (73,5)	11 (28,9)	0,0001
	No improvement	54 (26,5)	27 (71,1)	
Total		205 (100%)	38 (100%)	

There is a positive correlation between the post-test mark and the sum of the marks for the reasoning questions, with a correlation coefficient r =0.630, p<0.0001, r^2 =0.397.

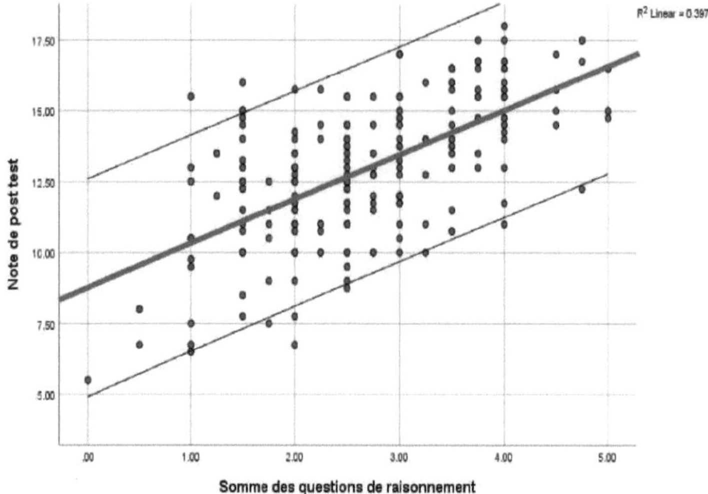

Figure 10: Scatterplot of post-test scores as a function of the sum of the reasoning questions.

d.   Correlation between the simulation score and the sum of the reasoning questions

There was a small but statistically significant correlation between the sum of the scores on the Level III reasoning questions and the score on the simulation exam.

(r=0.256, p<0.001, r2=0.066).

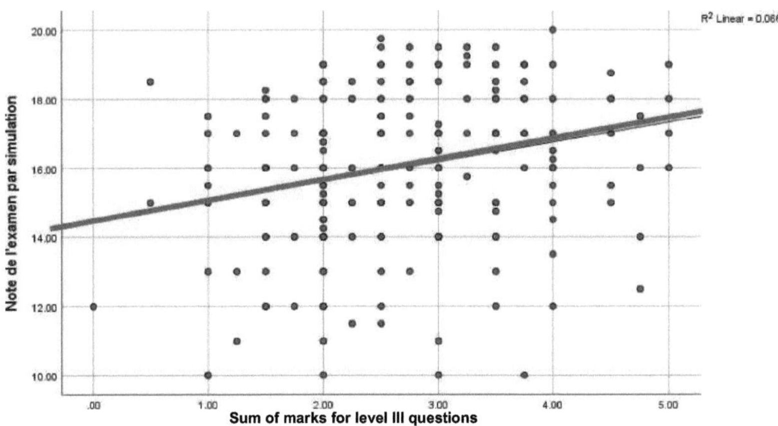

Figure 11: Scatter plot of simulated practice scores as a function of the sum of the reasoning questions

e. Correlation between simulation score and sum of post-test score, ANTS score and cardiac massage score

There is a strong, statistically significant correlation between the sum of the notes from the post-test examination, ANTS score, cardiac massage note and examination score by simulation. (r=**0.762**, p<0.001, r^2 =**0.581**).

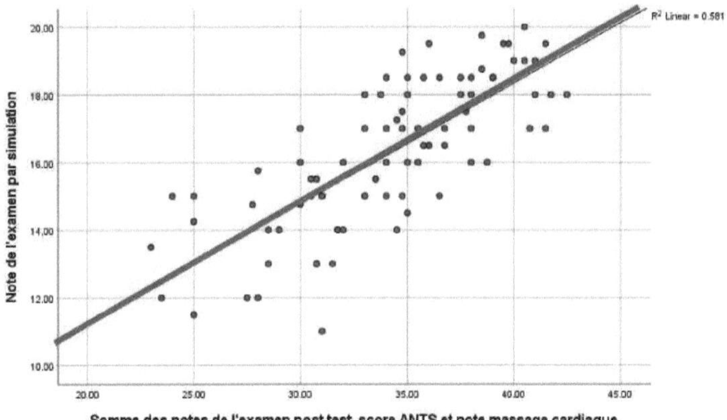

Figure 12: Scatter plot of the simulated practice score as a function of the sum of the scores for the knowledge questions, technical and non-technical gesture scores

Our study is considered to be the first carried out at the Sousse Faculty of Medicine, enabling an evaluation of the "CPR" module taught in the form of simulation-based learning to DCEM3 students during the 2022-2023 year.

The aim of our study was to evaluate the level of theoretical knowledge and technical and non-technical skills of DCEM3 students before and after simulation-based learning of the "Advanced CPR" module.

The results of our study showed that simulation-based training "in front of a patient in critical condition" was a teaching method appreciated by our learners. It enabled a statistically significant improvement in theoretical knowledge, as well as technical and non-technical knowledge, as it could affect the highest taxonomic levels.

Simulation therefore seems to be an essential tool for learning, because it initiates a systematisation of reflection on the action, enabling conceptualisation and transferability. It takes different forms and enables a variety of learning opportunities. The possibility of working on non-technical skills is one of the major advantages of these exercises (6).

The population of our study was represented by students of relatively young age, with an average of 23.6 (±0.7) and extremes ranging from 22-28.A clear female predominance (73%).

Kirkpatrick's first level is called "reaction". This level evaluates the learners' perception of the training and the method used, and implies learner satisfaction (4).

In our study, the overall impression of the CPR module was 92.4% between good and excellent, with more than half of the participants rating it as excellent. The participants were satisfied with the documents provided, the organisation of the session, the realism of the scenarios, the quality of the debriefing and the quality of the instructors' work.

By comparing them with the literature, our results were close to those obtained in

Tunisia by L. Bousoffara et al. in the Pneumology and Medical Intensive Care Departments of the Mahdia and Monastir Hospitals, from students who had taken part in high-fidelity simulation training sessions during their training period in pneumology. The majority of students (60%) were satisfied with the course of their training More than half judged the simulation sessions to be realistic (60%), compared with 52% who judged them to be excellent in our study (1).

another by Guillaume Der Sahakian et al at the University of Paris 5, Faculty of Medicine Paris-Descartes, used simulation as a means of learning and showed that the satisfaction of learners was good or excellent overall (100%)(7).

This proves that simulation is an effective means of motivating high-quality learning.

Learner satisfaction is of paramount importance and of great value in ensuring quality learning, but evaluation of the pedagogical impact alone remains unsatisfactory, which is why it must be supplemented by both theoretical and practical evaluation.

According to Kirkpatrick's model, the aim of the second "learning" level is to determine whether learners have acquired new knowledge, developed or improved their skills and changed their attitudes. Simulation therefore appears to be an essential tool for learning, as it initiates a systematisation of reflection on action, enabling conceptualisation and transferability(6).

In our study, learning was explored along two axes: theoretical knowledge and technical and non-technical skills.

The theoretical evaluation was carried out by means of a test completed by the students before and after the training course. In this test we tried to evaluate the different levels of knowledge, from simple cognitive to reasoning questions.

The median pre-test score was 9.5 [7.75 - 12], the median post-test score was 13 [14.75 - 11.5]. At the end of the CPR training day, 205 (84.4%) of the students improved their score. With a statistically significant difference (p<0.0001)

This improvement mainly concerned questions with a high taxonomic level requiring reasoning. We noted that 73.5% of learners who improved their score on the reasoning questions consequently improved their score on the post-test after the training session as well as their score on the final assessment (simulation scenario) with a significant difference (p<0.001).

This was in line with several other studies. Among others, the study by Fabien Beaufils et al in Poitiers, France in 2012 showed that the CPR knowledge of the childminder assessed by a questionnaire at the beginning and end of the session increased significantly after the didactic intervention on the management of infant cardiac arrest, the order of CPR steps, chest compression, ventilation and the emergency call(8).

Another experimental study carried out on medical students at a university in Brazil in 2018 showed that for most items, these students obtained a significant gain (P < 0.05) compared with the pre-test(9).

In the same context, another study carried out in 2017 by Joris Galland at Tenon Hospital with first-year DES interns revealed that 83% of participants acquired new theoretical knowledge following simulation-based training (10).

Similarly, another study carried out at the University of Paris Descartes in France revealed that simulation enables an improvement in knowledge that is complementary to experience, following an understanding of the obstacles linked to the implementation of theoretical knowledge (11).

A number of studies have demonstrated the value of simulation for learning technical procedures, particularly in the field of emergency medicine and intensive care anaesthesia (12).one of the advantages of simulation on a mannequin is that it enables training in the most common procedures (external cardiac massage) as well as those with much rarer indications (intercricothyroid puncture, thoracostomy, etc.).

In our study, we chose to evaluate an essential technical skill for extreme emergencies that all medical students must master: external cardiac massage (ECM). This evaluation enabled us to see the added value of this teaching method for learning practical skills.

The management of cardiac arrest requires mastery of a large number of technical techniques. Simulation enables each of these techniques to be practised under realistic conditions and repeated until they are learned. The rate and depth of chest compressions are two technical parameters associated with the prognosis of RCA that are extremely difficult to master(3).

In our study, the quality of cardiac massage was assessed using a 13-item grid(13). We showed an improvement in the students' marks; (69.8%) significantly improved their cardiac massage technique on the day of the examination (p<0.001).

Procedural simulation reproduces a part of the human body to learn a specific, more or less invasive gesture. In this same framework a quasi-experimental study was conducted at the Faculty of Medical Sciences in Shoushtar (IRAN) in September 2018 showed that simulation training of a vaginal delivery (VB) increased

significantly improved the performance of students in normal childbirth in a real environment during the training period(14) Another study carried out by Guillaume Der Sahakian et al at the University of Paris 5, Faculty of Medicine Paris-Descartes, with interns showed that the technical skills of interns assessed during several scenarios showed a significant increase of 46% (7).

A literature review of studies evaluating high-fidelity simulation in midwifery carried out in 2020 as part of a dissertation for the midwifery state diploma at Claude Bernard University - Lyon 1, using the PRISMA method, concluded that there was a significant improvement in the skills of the group trained by simulation in terms of dexterity and efficiency of manoeuvres (whether in neonatal resuscitation, managing PPH or shoulder dystocia during childbirth (12)).

The terms technical and non-technical skills are closely linked to healthcare simulation, but non-technical skills, which are supposed to encompass all relational, attitudinal and communication skills, are more complex to define (15). In our study, non-technical skills were assessed using the ANTS scale, which is based on 4 items, and is divided into 15 elements, each containing examples of behaviour (16)

Simulation isn't just about teaching technical skills. Using this learning method, we can put our learners in real-life situations and teach them to work as part of a team, communicate and understand leadership.

Our study showed a significant improvement in non-technical skills scores on the day of the exam (89.5%), with average scores ranging from 6.4 to 10.2.

Simulation improves communication between carers and between carers and patients. For example, the announcement of an illness or bad news has been the subject of several studies, which have shown the value of simulation for communicating this type of information to the patient (11).

This was also demonstrated by Richard et al, who showed the improvement and mastery of participants' crisis resource management (CRM) skills, as well as a good understanding of these skills during the debriefing. Of the nine self-reported CRM performance criteria studied, all reported an improvement in their non-technical CRM skills(17). Jason .Y et al, also showed the additional contribution of simulation-based team training in urology. Residents evaluated the simulation-based team training scenario as useful for training interdisciplinary communication skills (18) Simulation plays a crucial role in medical education by offering practical and innovative learning opportunities. It enables multidisciplinary exchanges and collaborations, promoting the development of projects between different simulation centres, offers unlimited pedagogical possibilities even with limited resources, improving teaching for medical students.

The integration of simulation into medical education is improving the licensing process, certification and the quality of patient care, thereby contributing to patient safety. Compared to flight simulators for pilots, its role has become essential in learning by doing in medicine and healthcare.

The limitations of our study were the small sample size and the fact that it was based on a single cohort, which could lead to a selection bias; moreover, it was a study concerned only with Kirkpatrick levels 1 and 2 patient care.

Nevertheless, our study was the first in our institution to assess the quality of simulation-based learning by studying the relationship between simulation and theoretical and practical knowledge, as well as the learning curve of medical students at different taxonomic levels. Simulation-based training offers medical students a safe and controlled environment in which to practise advanced techniques (CPR) without putting real patients at risk, improving knowledge acquisition, decision-making and performance compared with traditional teaching methods. This is why medical schools have incorporated it as a complement to traditional teaching methods, in order to contribute to the development of competent future doctors. However, it has its limitations in terms of cost and implementation.

Through our study, simulation appears to be an essential tool for learning, because it initiates a systematisation of reflection on action, enabling conceptualisation and transferability. It takes different forms and enables a variety of learning experiences. Simulation is a powerful tool for teaching and assessing CNT in medical students. Its growing use in medical training attests to its importance for the future of our healthcare systems. Our study showed a significant improvement in students' non-technical skills on the day of the examination. Simulation enhances communication between healthcare professionals and between them and patients, particularly in sensitive situations such as breaking bad news. It also improves crisis resource management skills and interdisciplinary communication. Similar to flight simulators for pilots, simulation plays a crucial role in practical learning in medicine and healthcare, offering numerous educational opportunities even with limited resources. Its integration into medical training improves accreditation and certification processes, enhancing the overall quality of patient care.

Simulation is a teaching method for acquiring and/or optimising a number of skills, such as communication, teamwork and theoretical knowledge. The opportunity to work on non-technical skills is one of the major benefits of these exercises. It is an essential means of maintaining patient safety by limiting the risk of errors. Simulation in the medical field is a learning method that is increasingly being developed in the specialities of acute care.

Numerous studies show that simulation significantly improves non-technical skills (NTS) in medical students, with a positive impact on patient safety. Its contribution to the development of competent future doctors who are concerned about patient safety is undeniable. It remains a powerful tool for teaching and assessing CNT in medical students. Its increasing use in medical training attests to its importance for the future of our healthcare systems. Our study showed a significant improvement in students' non-technical skills on the day of the examination. Simulation enhances communication between healthcare professionals and between them and patients, particularly in sensitive situations such as breaking bad news. It also improves crisis resource management skills and interdisciplinary communication.

The aim is therefore to promote this educational learning tool, particularly for medical students in their final year as externs, in an attempt to prepare them to deal with real-life situations in their internship sites.

Perspectives: Through our study, we have tried to evaluate Kirkpatrick's levels 1 and 2. The challenge remains to evaluate the third level, called "transfer", which enables us to assess the changes and modifications in the behaviour of learners in their work environment, and the fourth level, called "result", which enables us to identify the impact of simulation training on patient management.

REFERENCES

1. The contribution of simulation-based learning to the teaching of pulmonology - ScienceDirect [Internet]. [cited 7 Oct 2023]. Available from: https://www.sciencedirect.com/science/article/abs/pii/S07618425193107707 via %3Dihub

2. THE ROLE OF SIMULATION IN LEARNING CARDIAC ARREST RESUSCITATION IN 5TH YEAR MEDICAL STUDENTS - Google Search [Internet]. [cited 10 Oct 2023]. Available from: https://www.google.com/search?sca_esv=572214004&rlz=1C1GCEA_enTN 89 9TN899&sxsrf=AM9HkKky0gLICxsXGEwsNK-vlIkovmyABA: 1696950672062&q=PLACE+OF+SIMULATION+IN+L%27APPRENTISS AGE+IN+L%E2%80 %99CARDIATE+ARRET+FOR+STUDENTS+OF+5+EME+ANN EE+MEDICINE+THE+ROLE+OF+SIMULATION+IN+LEARNING+CAR D IAC+ARREST+RESUSCITATION+IN+5TH+YEAR+MEDICAL+STUDE NT   S&spell=   1 &sa=X&ved=2ahUKEwjZq4nw4euBAxUhTKQEHYrHDkIQBSgAe gQICBAB&cshid=1696950830707905&biw=1440&bih=789&dpr=1

3. Drummond D. Learning by simulation in paediatrics: the example of cardiorespiratory arrest in children. Ann Fr Médecine D'urgence. 1 Jul 2019;9(4):254-60.

4. 23-2010lelouarn-pottiez.pdf.

5. Ung N. Simulation en santé : état des lieux et mise en place pratique. Prat En Anesth Réanimation [Internet]. 14 Nov 2023 [cited 21 Nov 2023]; Available from:

https://www.sciencedirect.com/science/article/pii/S1279796023001468

6. Masson E. Intérêt pédagogique de la simulation [Internet]. EM-Consulte. [cited 10 Oct 2023]. Available from: https://www.em-consulte.com/article/1079797/interet-pedagogique-de-la-simulation

7. Guillaume DER SAHAKIAN, Lecomte FRANÇOIS, Kansao J, Grégory CARDOT, Kierzek G, Boubaker H, Claessens YE, Jean-Louis POURRIAT. Training interns in emergency medicine: simulation, an essential link? - Google Search [Internet]. [cited 4 May 2024]. Available from: https://www.google.com/search?q=Guillaume+DER+SAHAKIAN%2C+Lec om te+FRAN%C3%87OIS%2C+Kansao+J%2C+Gr%C3%A9gory+CARDOT% 2C +Kierzek+G%2C+Boubaker+H%2C+Claessens+YE%2C+Jean-Louis+POURRIAT.+Formation+des+internes+en+m%C3%A9decine+d%E 2% 80%99urgence+%3A+la+simulation%2C+un+maillon+indispensable+%3F &rlz =1C1 GCEA_enTN899TN899&oq=Guillaume+DER+SAHAKIAN%2C+Leco mte+FRAN%C3%87OIS%2C+Kansao+J%2C+Gr%C3%A9gory+CARDOT %2 C+Kierzek+G%2C+Boubaker+H%2C+Claessens+YE%2C+Jean-Louis+POURRIAT.+Formation+des+internes+en+m%C3%A9decine+d%E 2% 80%99urgence+%3A+la+simulation%2C+un+maillon+indispensable+%3F &aq s=chrome..69i57.1439j0j15&sourceid=chrome&ie=UTF-8

8. Beaufils F, Ghazali A, Boudier B, Gustin-Moinier V, Oriot D. Nursery Assistants' Performance and Knowledge on Cardiopulmonary Resuscitation: Impact of Simulation-Based Training. Front Pediatr. 2020;8:356.

9. Silva NL de C, de Melo M do CB, Liu PMF, Campos JPR, Arruda M de A. Teaching basic life support for medical students: Assessment of learning and

knowledge retention. J Educ Health Promot. 2023;12:218.

10. Simulation en santé : 1 re expérience en D.E.S de médecine interne | Request PDF [Internet]. [cited 4 May 2024]. Available from:

https://www.researchgate.net/publication/321437322_Simulation_en_sante_1_r e_experience_in_DES_internal_medicine

11. Hawkins A, Tredgett K. Use of high-fidelity simulation to improve communication skills regarding death and dying: a qualitative study. BMJ Support Palliat Care. Dec 2016;6(4):474-8.

12. The contribution of simulation to the management of life-threatening emergencies - Google Search [Internet]. [cited 4 May 2024]. Available from: https://www.google.com/search?q=Apport+of+simulation+for+taking+in+ch arge+of+vital+emergencies&rlz=1C1GCEA_enTN899TN899&oq=Contribu tion+of+simulation+for+taking+in+charge+of+vital+emergencies&aqs=chro me..69i57j69i60.1513j0j15&sourceid=chrome&ie=UTF -8

13. 2015NICEM013.pdf.

14. Pajohideh ZS, Mohammadi S, Keshmiri F, Jahangirimehr A, Honarmandpour A. The effects of normal vaginal birth simulation training on the clinical skills of midwifery students: a quasi-experiment study. BMC Med Educ. 19 May 2023;23(1):353.

15. Couarraze S, Saint-Jean M, Marhar F, Geeraerts T. Simulation in healthcare, a pedagogical tool vector of change in quality of life at work for anaesthesia resuscitation anaesthesia professionals. 2016.

16. Moll-Khosrawi P, Kamphausen A, Hampe W, Schulte-Uentrop L, Zimmermann S, Kubitz JC. Anaesthesiology students' Non-Technical skills: development and evaluation of a behavioural marker system for students (AS-NTS). BMC Med Educ. 13 June 2019;19(1):205.

17. Blum RH, Raemer DB, Carroll JS, Sunder N, Felstein DM, Cooper JB. Crisis resource management training for anaesthesia faculty: a new approach to continuing education. Med Educ. Jan 2004;38(1):45-55.

18. Lee JY, Mucksavage P, Canales C, McDougall EM, Lin S. High Fidelity Simulation Based Team Training in Urology: A Preliminary Interdisciplinary Study of Technical and Nontechnical Skills in Laparoscopic Complications Management. J Urol. Apr 2012;187(4):1385-91.

APPENDICES

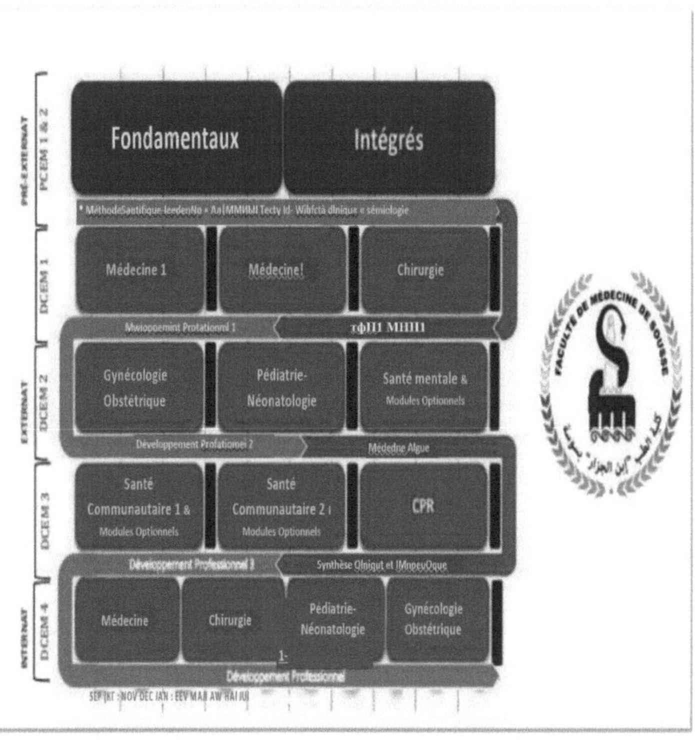

PRÉ-EXTERNAT
PCEM 1 & 2
Fondamentaux
Intégrés
DCEM 1
Méthode Santifique-leeden No » Au| MMИMI Tecty Id- Wibfctà dinique « sémiologie
Médecine 1
Médecine!
Chirurgie
EXTERNAT
DCEM 2
Mwioppemint Protationml 1
тФIII MIIII1
Gynécologie Obstétrique
Pédiatrie-Néonatologie
Santé mentale & Modules Optionnels
DCEM 3
Développement Profationei 2
Médecine Aigue
Santé Communautaire 1 & Modules Optionnels
Santé Communautaire 2 Modules Optionnels
CPR
INTERNAT
DCEM 4
Développement Professionnel 3
Synthèse Olnigut et IMnpevOque
Médecine
Chirurgie
Pédiatrie-Néonatologie
Gynécologie Obstétrique
1-
Développement Professionnel
SEP |KT : NOV DEC IAN : EEV MAI AW HAI JUI
FACULTÉ DE MÉDECINE DE SOUSSE

Nom ....   Prénom.................

Age...........................

Bonjour chers étudiants , vous êtes invités à répondre à ce questionnaire considéré comme un pré et un post est , qui s'introduit dans le cadre d'un travail de recherche se déroulant l'échelle institutionnelle , pour essayer d'évaluer « l'Apport de l'apprentissage par simulation dans la réanimation cardio pulmonaire avancé pour les étudiants en médecine sous graduer » comme nous sommes actuellement à la 3ème cohorte de notre faculté, vous avez eu votre support de cours théorique sur la plateforme, vous êtes appelés à répondre à ce questionnaire secondairement vous allez pratiquer tout au long de cette journée des différents « workshops » faisant répondre à des objectifs techniques et non techniques , on va vous noter sur ses compétences ainsi que sur le pré et post test pour essayer de dresser la courbe d'apprentissage ainsi que les différents niveaux d'apprentissage qu' on peut toucher avec cette nouvelle approche .

(NB que la note de ce teste ne fait pas partie de votre note d'examen final)

Si vous acceptez de participer, veuillez répondre à ce questionnaire

Merci

Evaluation des connaissances CPR 2023

1- **Pendant la réanimation cardio-pulmonaire avancée à l'hôpital :**
   a. un rapport de 5 ventilations pour 15 compressions cardiaques est correct
   b. la vérification d'une respiration normale ne doit pas durer plus de 10 secondes
   c. les mains devraient être positionnées sur le tiers supérieur du sternum pour réaliser les compressions thoraciques
   d. un coup de poing précordial peut être donné lors d'un arrêt par fibrillation ventriculaire devant témoin et monitoré
   e. des insufflations bouche à bouche sont recommandées

2- Vous arrivez 4 minutes après arrêt cardiaque chez une femme de 70 kg. Un accès IV est en place et il n'y a pas de pouls. L'ECG confirme une asystolie. Deux infirmières effectuent une RCP de manière efficace. Vous recommandez :
   a. administration d'un choc 360 J
   b. bicarbonate de sodium 500 mmol IV
   c. chlorure de calcium 5 ml solution 10% IV
   d. adrénaline 1 mg IVD.
   e. administrer de la cordarorne 300 mg en ivd

3- **Enumérer les différents rythmes choquables qu' on peut trouver lors d'un ACR**

4. **Au cours de la gestion des voies aériennes**
a. La meilleure approche pour reconnaître l'obstruction des voies aériennes est la VEA (voir/écouter/aspirer)
b. La libération des voies aériennes se base sur l'aspiration /mettre une canule oropharyngée
c. La canule doit être introduite rapidement dans la bouche du patient indépendamment de la taille
d. On peut utiliser comme moyen supra glottique le tube laryngé, le masque laryngé, et l'IGel
e. La perméabilité des voies aériennes et la ventilation des poumons sont des composants important à la ventilation

5- Pour le monitoring du rythme cardiaque :
   a. une fréquence ventriculaire de 60 à 100 pulsations/min est considérée normale
   b. une asystolie se présente comme un tracé complètement plat
   c. La fréquence cardiaque est calculée en divisant le nombre de grands carrés entre 2 ondes R par 60
   d. une tachycardie ventriculaire va toujours nécessiter une Cardioversion immédiate
   e. pour analyser un tracé électrique on doit répondre au minimum à 6 questions

6- La prise en charge correcte d'un patient adulte en FV comprend : DE

   a. digoxine 500 µg IV
   b. 1 mg d'adrénaline après chaque choc
   c. 3 mg d'atropine après deux boucles de RCP
   d. un choc initial bi phasique avec une énergie maximale 200j
   e. 300 mg de cordaronne en association avec le 3è CEE si persistance de la FV

7- Les compressions thoraciques :

   a. ne doivent pas être interrompues pour vérifier le pouls sauf si le patient montre des signes de vie
   b. deviennent en continue après une intubation orotrachéale
   c. devrait être effectuées à un rythme de 60/minute pour les adultes
   d. devraient être commencées pour tout patient inconscient
   e. Le temps de compression égal au temps de décompression

8- monsieur MN de 56 tabagiques <u>actif</u>, s'est présenté aux urgences pour une douleur thoracique à l'examen il a perdu conaissance, le tracé électrique lors du monitorage du patient était comme suit :

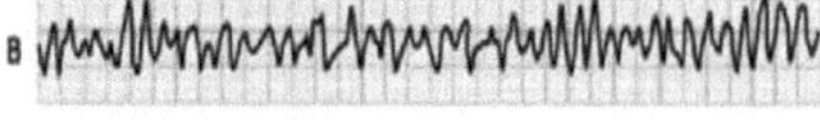

Décrire votre conduite à tenir immédiate

9- L'approche ABCDE
    a) Permet une évaluation rigoureuse d'un patient présentant un ACR
    b) Est une évaluation clinique où l'appréciation des voies aériennes libres et sures représente le « B »
    c) Est une approche au cours de laquelle il faut toujours faire une évaluation de l'état du patient suivie d'une action
    d) Consiste à faire un examen clinique complet d'un patient en état critique et le réévaluer régulièrement
    e) Travailler en équipe mais sans retour d'informations et sans communication

10- Au cours d'une réanimation cardio pulmonaire :
    a. le rythme doit être vérifié toute les 5 min
    b. Il faut toujours penser aux causes réversibles
    c. Il faut arrêter le massage cardiaque pour identifier le rythme
    d. On doit traiter les causes réversibles
    e. L'intubation orotrachéale du patient est primordiale

11. Mme S.D se présente aux urgences avec une FA rapide à 180 primo découverte, à l'examen elle présente une sat 92% avec une TA 09/60, des extrémités froides

Décrire votre conduite à tenir immédiate

12- Les (la) cause(s) réversible(s) recherché(es) :

a. Sont identifiés par les 5H et 5T
b. Peuvent être une hypoglycémie ; une hyperkaliémie ; un pneumothorax, une embolie pulmonaire ...
c. Nécessite(nt) parfois l'arrêt du massage cardiaque pour examiner le patient
d. Peut être une hypo volémie nécessitant une transfusion
e. Peut être une bradycardie nécessitant le recours à l'atropine

13- pour le bon déroulement d'une RCP

a. Il faut se répartir les tâches en fonction des compétences des intervenants
b. Le team leader doit contrôler le bon déroulement des instructions données au membre de son équipe
c. Les teams membres doit travailler en silence, chacun fait sa tâche discrètement
d. A la fin de la RCP toute l'équipe doit faire le débriefing pour en discuter les points à améliorer
e. Un team membre peut faire plus qu'une tache à la fois s'il est le plus compétent

14- monsieur M.N âgé de 65 ans diabétique sous ADO est arrivé aux urgences pour une douleur thoracique, brutalement il a présenté un ACR, après reconnaissance de l'ACR, on a identifié un BAV complet à 35c/min,

***Notre conduite à tenir est de :

a. Commencer immédiatement le massage cardiaque
b. Administrer immédiatement l'adrénaline à raison 1 mg en ivd
c. Administre un CEE avec une énergie maximale
d. Donner de l'atropine à raison de 0.5mg toute les 5 min
e. Chercher la cause le l'ACR avant d'administrer un traitement

***la RCP de monsieur M.N a duré 8min tout en gardant le même rythme, il a récupéré un pouls avec un rythme régulier sinusale :
a. Au cours de son RCP monsieur MN a reçu 4mg d'adrénaline
b. La cordaronne doit être administré dans le 3è cycle (6min)
c. Devant la douleur thoracique, on doit thrombolyser le patient pendant la RCP
d. Au cours de la RCP, on doit délivrer un CEE chaque fois que le rythme devient choquable
e. en post récupération, on doit évaluer le patient selon l'approche ABCDE

08:30-09 :00	Introduction		
09:00 - 09 :45	**Workshop: BLS and defibrillation**		
	Classe 1	Classe 2	Classe 3
09:45- 10:45	**Workshop :deteriorating Patient ABCDE**		
	Classe 1	Classe 2	Classe 3
10:45 - 11:00	Coffee/Tea		
11: 00- 11 :45	**Workshop: Airway &intraosseous access**		
	Classe 1	Classe 2	Classe 3
11:45 – 13:15	**Workshop: Rhythm/EKG Tachycardia-Cardioversion Bradycardia-Pacing**		
	Classe 1	Classe 2	Classe 3
13:15-13:30	**Lecture "ALS algorithm" :**		
13:30- 14:15	LUNCH		
14:15-14:45	**CAST Demo incl NTS**		
14:45-15:30	**CASTeach 1:shockable rhythms (SCA) +CASTeach 4 Post Resuscitation TSV**		
	Classe 1	Classe 2	Classe 3
15:30-16:15	**CASTeach2: Non-shockable rhythms (Hypovolaemia) +CASTeach 3 Decision making (asystolie) Trauma**		
	Classe 1	Classe 2	Classe 3
16:15 -17:00	**Special CircumstancesAnaphylaxia Asthma Electrolyte disorders**		
	Classe 1	Classe 2	Classe 3

Cesime FMS

Classe 1	
Classe 2	
Classe 3	

CESU CHU SAHLOUL

Classe 1	
Classe 2	
Classe 3	

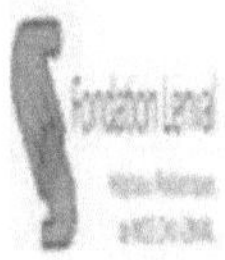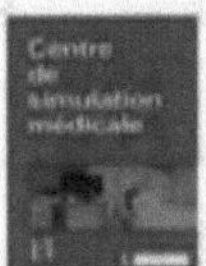

RESCAPE-CM

Evaluation du massage cardiaque du

adult

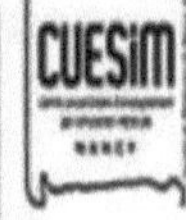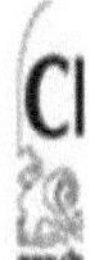

NOM	PRENOM

Yes(=I) No(=0)

	General principles		
HM-1	Massage method suitable for Γ Цe		
HM-2	Placing the child on a hard surface or massage board		
HM-3	Correct frequency (100-120/mm)		
HM-4	Ration compression /relaxation dtlïl___________		
HM-5	Rabo compression/ventilation dq 3o/2		
	Correct chest depression /1/3 of the domrtrp anttfü potitnturl		
HM-7	Step (f interruption of gesture		
	Cardiac massage from ⁊ᴘ ᴜ		
HM-8	Mum correctly positioned on the thorax (fobn on *b mo "t bfénture of the sternum*)		
HM-9	Fingers not resting on chest		
ИМ-10	Correct positioning of the rescuer /bterobment à b inrtme)		
им-II	Arms extended with elbows locked		
HM-12	Depression of thorax perpendicular to body tax		
HM-u	The heel of the hand does not lift off the chest during the relaxation phase		

Anesthesiologist's Nontechnical Skills (ANTS) Global Rating Scale

Subtopics	Elements	Partial Rating (1-4)	Global Category Rating (1-4)
Task Management			
	Planning and preparing		
	Prioritizing		
	Providing and maintaining standards		
	Identifying and utilizing resources		
Team Working			
	Coordinating activities with team		
	Exchanging information		
	Using authority and assertiveness		
	Assessing capabilities		
	Supporting others		
Situation Awareness			
	Gathering information		
	Recognizing and understanding		
	Anticipating		
Decision-making			
	Identifying options		
	Balancing risks and selecting options		
	Reevaluating		
	TOTAL POINTS (total of global ratings)		

-
-

Rating Options		Descriptor
Good	4	Performance was of a consistently high standard, enhancing patient safety; it could be used as a positive example for others
Acceptable	3	Performance was of a satisfactory standard but could be improved
Marginal	2	Performance indicated cause for concern, considerable improvement is needed
Poor	1	Performance endangered or potentially endangered patient safety, serious remediation is required

-
- Subject Number _____________   Date _____________

MODELE D'EVALUATION DE LA FORMATION DE KIRKPATRICK

47

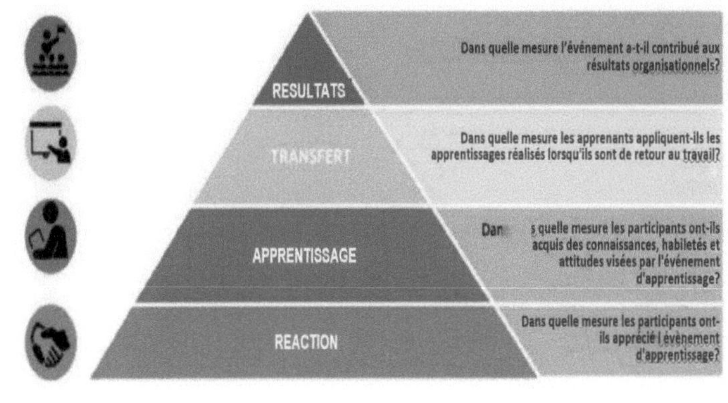

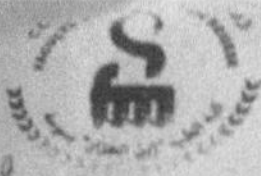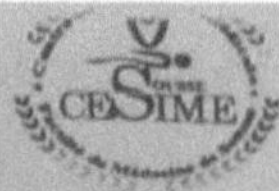

Université de Sousse
Faculté de médecine de Sousse
Centre de Simulation Médicale de Sousse

Date:................................Année d'étude:............................Titre de la séance:..............................

ÉVALUATION DE LA FORMATION PAR SIMULATION

Veuillez évaluer les différents éléments de ce programme de formation en utilisant l'échelle ci-dessous :

1 - Inadéquat	2 - Insuffisant	3 - Adéquat	4 - Bon	5 - Excellent

INTRODUCTION

	1	2	3	4	5
Document à lire	☐	☐	☐	☐	☐
Présentation de l'introduction	☐	☐	☐	☐	☐
Révision du vidéo déclencheur	☐	☐	☐	☐	☐
Orientation au simulateur	☐	☐	☐	☐	☐

Commentaires

ÉQUIPEMENTS ET ENVIRONNEMENT

	1	2	3	4	5
Organisation générale de la salle de simulation	☐	☐	☐	☐	☒
Mannequins	☐	☐	☐	☐	☒
Moniteur du patient	☐	☐	☐	☐	☒
Aide mémoire	☐	☐	☐	☐	☒
Médication fournie	☐	☐	☐	☐	☐
Équipement audiovisuel	☐	☐	☐	☐	☒
Réalisme général de l'environnement de simulation	☐	☐	☐	☐	☐

Commentaires

SCÉNARIOS

	1	2	3	4	5
Réalisme des scénarios	☐	☐	☐	☐	☒
Réalisme des indices visuels	☐	☐	☐	☒	☐
Réalisme des indices sonores	☐	☐	☐	☒	☐
Réalisme des indices tactiles	☐	☐	☐	☒	☐
Réalisme des acteurs ou patients partenaires dans les scénarios	☐	☐	☐	☐	☒
Capacité du scénario à faire valoir les habiletés techniques	☐	☐	☐	☐	☒
Capacité du scénario à faire valoir les attitudes et comportements	☐	☐	☐	☐	☒
Qualité générale des scénarios	☐	☐	☐	☐	☒

Commentaires

"DÉBRIEFING"

	1	2	3	4	5
Le " débriefing " a permis de clarifier certains éléments particuliers.	☐	☐	☐	☐	☒
Le " débriefing " a permis une rétroaction constructive.	☐	☐	☐	☒	☐
Le " débriefing " a permis de revoir les habiletés techniques démontrées.	☐	☐	☐	☒	☐
Le " débriefing " a permis de revoir les attitudes et comportements démontrés.	☐	☐	☐	☐	☒
Qualité générale du " débriefing "	☐	☐	☐	☐	☒

Commentaires

INSTRUCTEURS

	1	2	3	4	5
Les instructeurs ont créé un environnement d'apprentissage accueillant.	☐	☐	☐	☐	☒
Les instructeurs ont facilité le " débriefing ".	☐	☐	☐	☐	☒
Les instructeurs ont su créer des liens entre les scénarios et des cas réels.	☐	☐	☐	☐	☒
Enthousiasme des instructeurs	☐	☐	☐	☐	☒
Qualité générale du travail des instructeurs	☐	☐	☐	☒	☐
Est-ce que vous avez ressenti un conflit d'intérêt au biais ?	☒ non		☐ oui		

Commentaires

GÉNÉRAL

	1	2	3	4	5
Impression générale	☐	☐	☐	☐	☒

Quelles parties de l'atelier ou du programme ai-je le plus aimé ?

Quelles parties de l'atelier ou du programme ai-je le moins aimé ?

Qu'est-ce qui pourrait rendre cet atelier ou programme meilleur ?

Commentaires

ÍNDICE

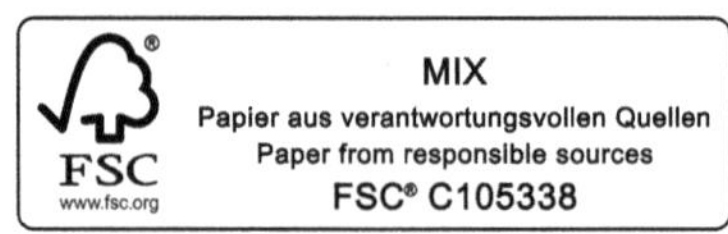

Printed by Books on Demand GmbH, Norderstedt / Germany